Polyvagal Theory

A Beginner's Guide to Discovering the Autonomic Nervous System and Understanding Stress, Depression and Anxiety

Erika Newton

Table of Contents

Introduction

C ustomarily the autonomic nervous system was perceived for its guideline of the different instinctive "programmed" capacities, for example, absorption, breath, sex drive, propagation, and so on. The old model of pressure or unwinding depended on perceiving just two circuits—the sympathetic and the parasympathetic. In the old model, the sympathetic nervous system was viewed as dynamic in stress reaction to dangers and risk. The parasympathetic nervous system, on the other hand, communicated in the unwinding reaction and was related to the capacity of the vagus nerve. This more established, all-around acknowledged model of the autonomic nervous system expected that there is a solitary vagus nerve, and it didn't assess the way that there are really two very unique neural pathways that are both called "vagus."

The Polyvagal Theory starts by perceiving that the vagus nerve has two separate branches—two discrete, particular vagal nerves that begin in two unique areas. We get a progressively exact portrayal of the operations of the autonomic nervous system. The autonomic nervous system comprises three neural circuits: the ventral branch of the vagus nerve (positive states of unwinding and social engagement), the spinal sympathetic chain (battle or flight), and the dorsal branch of the vagus nerve (slowdown, shutdown, and burdensome conduct). These three circuits direct our substantial capacities so as to assist our bodies with homeostasis.

The Polyvagal Theory likewise displays another measurement to our comprehension of the autonomic nervous system. The autonomic nervous system not just controls the capacity of our inward organs; these three circuits additionally identify with our emotional states, which thusly drive our conduct. Individuals who give massages know for a fact that one individual's body may be excessively tight, another may be excessively delicate, and a third can feel "perfect." Usually, when specialists are prepared to give a massage, they figure out how to discharge pressure in a strained muscle. Notwithstanding, this methodology doesn't take a shot at a body that needs adequate tone.

Movement bolstered by the spinal sympathetic chain empowers us to battle so as to meet danger head-on or flee to maintain a strategic distance from it. This is because hard, tense muscles allow us to move the whole body more rapidly. Worse hypertension is additionally expected to get the flow of blood into muscles that are strained and hard.

Low levels of muscle tonus are discovered when the dorsal vagal circuit is actuated when there is no compelling reason to tense the muscles to battle or escape (or, at times of outrageous threat, when the body's endurance reaction is too close down). Low blood pressure is adequate to get the blood into delicate, limp muscles. In its outrageous structure, this low blood pressure may make individuals lose cognizance and swoon. The restorative term for this is "syncope." Normal blood pressure is suitable for neither tense nor limp muscles. In states of social engagement, there is commonly no risk or threat in our condition or body. Our nervous system activates this reality, so we don't need to do anything; we can genuinely unwind and appreciate being with others. As far as the Polyvagal Theory, we can be immobilized, unafraid, outraged, or feel burdensome when we are in a condition of social engagement. Our blood pressure, blood sugar, and temperature are generally typical. We can stay composed yet wakeful and alert.

A handshake gives us a decent sign of the condition of someone else's autonomic nervous system. An excessively tight body, as a rule, results from an incessant condition of action in the spinal sympathetic chain, where the whole solid system is ceaselessly arranged to battle or escape. Such an individual typically has an excessively compelling handshake, pressing more earnestly than would normally be appropriate. The inverse is valid for somebody lacking strong tonus—generally an indication of over-movement in the dorsal vagal circuit. This individual, by and large, has a limp, moist, and, every now and then, chilly handshake. In the event that our handshake is perfect, it is the ventral branch of the vagus nerve that is transcendent. We may have a few pressures in individual muscles. However, the strained muscles loosen up rapidly, and a massage specialist will see that our body likewise feels right. The tonus of the muscles is just one of numerous approaches to screening the condition of the body's nervous system.

HOMEOSTASIS AND THE ANS

The neural circuits controlling the nerves managing instinctive organ capacity can be contrasted with an indoor regulator connected to both a warmer and a forced-air system. At the point when the indoor regulator enlists that the air is excessively chilly, it turns on the warmer, and if the air is excessively warm, it turns into a real-time conditioner. Warm-blooded creatures comparably need to keep up internal heat level within upper and lower limits, and their tactile nerves give criticism about internal heat level to their "indoor regulator."

Standards of conduct, just as physiological capacities, help the body to direct temperature. For instance, if we are cold, we can move around to create heat through the action of our muscles, or we can put on more garments to protect ourselves and reduce the loss of body heat. The blood vessels of the skin choke to save heat. When we are freezing, our bodies begin to shudder wildly, creating heat from the activity of the muscles. At the point when we are warm, we rest or sit still so as to diminish strong movement and, in this way, stay away from further overheating. The blood vessels enlarge, allowing more warmth to arrive at the skin surface, where it very well may be scattered. We take off layers of apparel, and we sweat; when our perspiration vanishes, it cools the body. At the point when individuals are irate, we now and then state that they are "angry as a mad bull." We may reprove them to "cool it." When individuals don't care for something, they may pull back, and we state that they are "cool" to it. We consider approaches to "warm them up" to the thought. Both warmth and coolness are detected as impressions of emotional states.

The three parts of the autonomic nervous system cooperate to control the action of the organs, realize homeostasis, and assist us with suitably meeting ecological circumstances and equalization conditions inside the body. We can likewise apply the model of the Polyvagal Theory to issues and findings in numerous physiological territories, for example, assimilation or proliferation, which we may somehow or another consider to be physical issues outside our ability to control or impact. For instance, a developing collection of logical research utilizes pulse changeability (HRV) to gauge ventral vagal movement by measuring an unconstrained beat in pulse known as respiratory sinus arrhythmia. These examinations locate that low degrees of ventral vagal action are connected to a wide scope of medical problems, for example, weight, hypertension, heart variances, and so on. There are likewise a few hypotheses that HRV is a possibly valuable estimation to help anticipate the beginning of a disease, malignant growth metastasis, or the reasonable mortality of individuals with diseases.

The Five States of the Autonomic Nervous System

BIOBEHAVIOR: THE INTERACTION OF BEHAVIOR AND BIOLOGICAL PROCESSES

In contrast to the old model of the autonomic nervous system, which concentrated only on its guideline of the capacity of the instinctive organs, the new model of the autonomic nervous system incorporates three particular neural pathways, as discussed above, and relates every one of these three neural circuits with a passionate state, which drives our conduct. Notwithstanding these three states, we have two half and half expresses, every one of which consolidates two of the individual circuits, for an aggregate of five potential states of our autonomic nervous system. One half and half state bolster the experience of closeness: the dorsal vagus is locked in to hinder our physical movement, simultaneously as the ventral vagus permits a sentiment of wellbeing with someone else. This is talked about in further detail beneath.

The subsequent half and half state communicate in a benevolent challenge. We may contend energetically to win in sports or games, yet this happens inside a system of security and rules to which the entirety of the rivals have concurred ahead of time. In this cross breed expression, the battle or flight reaction of spinal thoughtful chain initiation is joined with the sentiments of wellbeing related to the action of the ventral vagus branch.

THE THREE NEURAL PATHWAYS OF THE ANS

The first of the autonomic nervous system's neural pathways is the social commitment nervous system. It includes action in the ventral branch of the vagus nerve (CN X) and four other cranial nerves (CN V, VII, IX, and XI). Movement in this circuit has a quieting, relieving impact and advances rest and compensation. The ventral branch of the vagus nerve identifies with positive feelings of bliss, fulfillment, and love. When it comes to conduct, it communicates in positive social exercises with companions and friends, and family. The condition of social commitment bolsters social practices in which we back up and offer help to other individuals. Collaboration with others typically improves our odds for endurance—we talk together, sing together, move together, share a supper, coordinate to finish a task, instruct and sustain youngsters, and so on.

The second of the ANS's neural pathways is the spinal thoughtful chain, which is enacted when our endurance is undermined. In the event that we assemble our body with this reaction, we can attempt to assist us with reacting to the risk. This condition of "assembly with dread" emerges when we are not protected or don't have a sense of security. Condition of "activation with dread" emerges when we are not sheltered or don't have a sense of security. The spinal thoughtful chain identifies with feelings of outrage or dread, which can convey what needs to be in practice, for example, battling to defeat the danger or escaping to keep away from an undermining circumstance.

The third neural pathway is the dorsal branch of the vagus nerve. This pathway is actuated when we face a staggering power and up-and-coming annihilation. When there is no reason for battling or fleeing, we moderate what assets we have—we immobilize. Actuation of this pathway cultivates sentiments of vulnerability, misery, and lack of care showing in withdrawal and shutdown. This state can be portrayed as "immobilization with dread." When people or different well-evolved creatures are looked at with apparently inescapable human threat, demise, or devastation, the dorsal branch of our vagus nerve is initiated. An abrupt or outrageous flood of dorsal vagal action can offer ascent to a condition of stun or shutdown. Among different reactions, the solid system loses its tonus, and the pulse drops. We may black out or go into a condition of stun (syncope).

Natural life documentaries on the African fields have caught the accompanying scene. A lion pursues and catches a baby antelope and takes it up in its forceful jaws. The baby antelope had been in a condition of spinal thoughtful chain action when it was undermined and fled. Presently, confronting fast approaching passing, it goes into stun and shutdown: it swoons, and its body goes limp. Lions are not by and large foragers. On the off chance that a lion all of a sudden develops faculties that tell it that its prey has gotten dormant, it might open its jaws, drop the prey, and move away. Exactly when the lion is going to shake the baby antelope to break its neck or dive into its tissue, the limp muscles neglect to give the typical obstruction. Maybe the antelope's shutdown reaction is sufficient to invalidate the lion's executioner impulse. The lion discharges its grasp, the baby antelope tumbles to the ground, and the lion moves away.

A few moments after the lion leaves, the baby antelope stands up, shakes it off, and returns to its mom. It, at that point, resumes touching as though nothing has occurred. The baby antelope is prepared to confront the following to test its endurance because of its lifesaving shutdown reaction. This represents the versatile endurance estimation of the dorsal-branch immobilization reaction in circumstances of outrageous risk. We see another case of how the dorsal branch of the vagus nerve can encourage a fruitful barrier: A porcupine, confronting peril from a predator, pulls back by folding up into a ball. Its sharp plumes fiber out-ward, making it next to impossible for the predator to effectively nibble it.

The Two-Hybrid Circuits

Notwithstanding these three circuits of the autonomic nervous system, there are two hybrid states comprised of various mixes of two of the three neural circuits. The fourth state is a hybrid that supports benevolent challenge, or "preparation unafraid," which is there for when we take part in aggressive games. This state joins the impacts of two neural circuits: enactment of the spinal thoughtful chain enables us to assemble ourselves to accomplish our best execution. Actuation of the social commitment circuit keeps things cordial, so we can play securely inside the guidelines and abstain from harming one another.

In sports, we can contend energetically to win. The two groups consent to observe the guidelines and remain within limits to protect

11

everything. All things considered, it is just a game. There are numerous different instances of activating bravery. Young doggies from a similar litter always play with one another as though they were battling. They snarl and chomp each other for a considerable length of time.

The fifth state is additionally a hybrid of two neural circuits. Action in the dorsal part of the vagus nerve, when joined with that of the ventral part of the vagus nerve, underpins sentiments of closeness and private conduct. This state, which we could call "immobilization unafraid," is described as a quiet that confides in sentiments, permitting us, for instance, to lie still and nestle with a friend or family member.

NOTES

Chapter 1:
The Evolution of Polyvagal Theory

A t the point when I began my logical profession, I was interested in the plausibility of utilizing physiological measures to comprehend the mental conditions of others. In the late 1960s, when I was in graduate school, I had the vision that observing a physiological state would be a useful manual for the advisor during clinical communication. This vision is still a piece of my inquire about motivation. I am as yet taking a shot at building up a polyvagal screen, which will give input progressively to clinicians of the dynamic interchange between the three neural circuits depicted in the polyvagal theory.

During the 1960s, the developments and models relating physiology to conduct were constrained. Prevailing in human and psychophysiological writing was a build of excitement. The characterizing highlights of excitement were dubious. In any case, psychophysiologists expected that the thoughtful apprehensive framework intervened arousal. Early psychophysiologists, for example, Chester Darrow, proposed coherence between cortical initiation estimated through electroencephalography (EEG), what's more, thoughtful excitement estimated by the galvanic skin obstruction reaction on the hands. This perspective on a fringe marker of mind forms was reliable with Pavlov's utilization of autonomic measures in his traditional molding tests. For Pavlov, the "traditionally" molded autonomic reactions were lists of changes in cerebrum circuits. Excitement is as yet utilized in the rest of the research to portray cortical enactment and inquire about the trickery in which customary polygraphs are utilized. The particular physiological and neurophysiological components of basic excitement are regularly connected with the thoughtful sensory system and the hypothalamic-pituitary-adrenal (HPA) hub. An induced association between the thoughtful sensory system and the HPA pivot has brought about comparative research strategies being utilized to think about both excitement and stress. This thoughtful, driven view has been converted into the mainstream press and open cognizance as an antique that a restricted measure of pressure is "great," and an excess of stress is "terrible." But what were the limits of pressure important for wellbeing or disease? What's more, reliable with this sympathetic-centric view, we as a whole were instructed that the stress-related thoughtful excitation had transformative causes in mammalian fight or flight practices. In this way, we were instructed that the expanded thoughtful tone of oddity and threat was an impression of our developmental history.

The polyvagal theory is a comprehension of the reiteration of our developmental history. For well-evolved creatures, the developmental history is really called phylogeny, which deals with the sensory systems (or their highlights) that we've acquired from our precursors. For this situation, the predecessors are reptiles, land, and water proficient, furthermore, fish. As vertebrates, we have acquired a lot of circuits. As these circuits transform, they brought about utilitarian neuro-stages for a large number of the practices we as people express. One thing we have overlooked or didn't comprehend until the polyvagal theory empowered us to have the reconceptualization was our extraordinary progress from reptiles to warm-blooded animals. In that progress from old reptiles to even the crude warm-blooded animals, certain things happened. Those things are tied in with empowering co-guideline in a sense, empowering one well-evolved creature to help direct the physiological condition of another well-evolved creature. That required prompting, or the social commitment, of another with signals of wellbeing and signs of security to empower two of the species to be agreeable in one another's essence.

The entire history of warm-blooded creatures is tied in with being agreeable within sight of another proper warm-blooded animal. It's truly what gets disturbed with injury. At the point when an injury happens, individuals are never again ready to cohabitate with another, since regularly the injury has been delivered by another person and their sensory system presently doesn't welcome the other individual into their quality. The polyvagal model truly has three polyvagal states, including the crudest framework that we've acquired, which is imparted to for all intents and purposes all vertebrates. It returns to the ligament that fish have, which is identified with the capacity to immobilize with dread and utilize fixed status as a guard framework. This becomes one of the basic focuses – that is, people who have gone into a breakdown or a demise faking have changed on the grounds that they've obtained access to this extremely old knowledge. Hereditarily, the following stage that developed was the assembly framework, which we as a whole know as battle flight. In any case, battle flight likewise has certain magnificent points of interest, since as long as we continue moving, we're not going to be defenseless against closed down or breakdown. You see those side effects in numerous individuals who have injury chronicles.

Being in a physiological condition of battle flight isn't awesome for one's body. It prompts ailments. It's additionally shocking for social communications since we need to sign others to, as it were, remain quiet, co-control, and offer encounters. We could utilize the term between abstract encounters. We need to share contemplations and thoughts and all things considered to be available with another. With the appearance of warm-blooded animals, a more up-to-date circuit went ahead, and this is what we're naming either the ventral vagal circuit or the social commitment framework. The social commitment framework was really connecting the neuro-guideline of all the muscles, the strident muscles that control the face and head – including the muscles of vocalization, the muscles of tuning in, the muscles of prompting in the face, also, the muscles of how we articulate the prosodic highlights in our voice with the vagal guideline of the heart.

We fundamentally are continually wearing our face on our heart, and we're passing on our physiological state in our voice. We are identifying the physiological condition of others through their voices and with their countenances. When we watch somebody, we get signals from the speaker's face, tuning in to their voice and choosing if this is an agreeable individual to listen to. Or on the other hand, whether or not I should consider the words or if it would be a good idea for me to consider the sentiments that the words pass on. So the social commitment framework is truly what makes people human or really makes a warm-blooded creature's vertebrate.

The social commitment framework is this superb capacity to pass on to another what our physiological state is. What the polyvagal theory assembles is the view that these circuits are progressive. Progressive implies that more up-to-date circuits have the ability to restrain the more seasoned ones. This means social commitment can down-manage battle flight and can quiet us down similarly as a battle flight can keep us out of closing down. There are three levels, and everyone represses the more crude framework underneath it. The word that was utilized to portray this is a word called "disintegration," which originates from researcher John Hughlings Jackson, who was exceptionally intrigued by cerebrum forms and in this hindrance of mind circuits, with the goal that they become more crude and receptive when we have cerebrum harm or ailment. So the autonomic sensory system works a similar way. Our most up-to-date circuit quiets us; our more seasoned circuits can be utilized for safeguard.

What enables social commitment to happen while the guarded systems of fight-flight are being debilitated? Stephen utilizes the expression "include identifiers" that essentially expect that our sensory system developed to identify includes in the other, to assist us with distinguishing wellbeing. So those component finders are a piece of the build he calls "neuroception." You can't talk about the social commitment framework without discussing neuroception. Neuroception is the instrument through which our sensory system identifies wellbeing and afterward empowers the social commitment framework to work. It distinguishes this without mindfulness. It is a unique framework since it isn't the subjective mindfulness we are in a safe environment.

Our sensory system is identifying the degree of security; at that point, the physiology reacts. One can be extremely mindful of their physiology. Much like setting off to an address, we go in, and we state, "Well, the words sound great or if nothing else if I somehow managed to understand it, it would be great, however you know, there is something in particular about that individual that I don't generally feel great with." Everyone has had those issues. It is difficult to mark; however, we feel awkward; perhaps it's an absence of prosody in that individual's voice, the absence of commitment. We could state it is the absence of being extremely delicate or then again having the feeling that the other is being a substantial individual. It's actually that the words are there, yet the emotions underneath the words may not be. That is the thing that our bodies are reacting to. We react more significantly to the lessening of voice than we do to what is said by the individual. When our body reacts, we feel it and afterward build up our very own story. That is the way we either feel that we can be near individuals, or we feel that we ought to be truly separating. The hidden topic here is, there is no social commitment, except if our neuroception gets the highlights of security.

NOTES

Chapter 2:
The Vagus Nerve

T he vagus nerve is known as the longest and most complex of the 12 pairs of cranial nerves, and it originates from the brain. It is in charge of the transmission of information to or from the brain to tissues and organs connected in the body.

It was originally cited as "pneumogastric" before the name "vagus," which came from the Latin term which literally means "wandering," was adopted. This is because the vagus nerve has the longest and most diverse pathway around the body, and it is believed, it "wanders" into tissues and organs in the neck, chest, and abdomen from the brain.

It is the 10th cranial nerve and thus known as the "10th cranial nerve" or "cranial nerve X."

The vagus nerve has sensory nerve cell bodies that come in two bunches, and it serves as a connection between the brainstem (from which it originates) to the body (to which it extends to). It allows the brain to receive information and monitor several of the body's different organic and tissue functions.

The vagus is a mixed nerve that contains parasympathetic fibers carrying somatic and visceral afferents and efferents.

The majority of fibers of the vagus nerve are visceral afferents because of the vast nature of cutting across the thoracic and abdominal cavity, and its internal organs such as the heart, lungs, stomach, gut, etc., and they have a wide distribution that can pass through the central nervous system (CNS). This passage occurs either through the nucleus of the sole tract or monosynaptically. Aside from stimulation of well-defined reflexes, vagus nerve activation produces the manifestation of potentials recorded from the cerebral cortex, the hippocampus, the thalamus, and the cerebellum.

The terminating part of the vagus nerve is called the spinal accessory nucleus.

Etymology

Vagus is a Latin word that means "wandering." It originates from the same root as "vagabond," "vagrant," "divagation," and "vague."

The vagus nerve is most times described in singular terms even though it is paired but sometimes the right and left branches together are called off in the plural as vagi (/ ˈveɪdʒaɪ/ VAY-jy).

The vagus was once historically called the pneumogastric nerve since it was known to be in charge of innervating both the lungs and the stomach.

Structure

Originating from the medulla oblongata, the vagus nerve runs between the pyramid (olive) and the inferior cerebellar peduncle; it extends through the jugular foramen, then passes into the carotid sheath, which is between the internal carotid artery and the internal jugular vein down to the neck, thorax, and abdomen, where it makes contributions to the innervation of the viscera, extending all the way to the colon. That is the reason why it is the longest and most complex of all 12 cranial nerves.

Aside from giving some output to various organs as efferent functions, the vagus nerve is made up of between 80% to 90% of afferent nerves, mostly transmitting sensory information about the state and wellbeing of the body's organs to the central nervous system (CNS).

The vagus nerve comes in a pair; the right and the left vagus nerves, and they descend from the cranial vault passing through the jugular foramina into the carotid sheath, which is between the internal and external carotid arteries, then extends posterolaterally to the common carotid artery. The cell bodies of the vagal visceral afferent fibers are found bilaterally in the inferior vagus nerve ganglia (nodose ganglia).

The right vagus nerve ascends into the neck between the trachea and esophagus when it gives rise to the right recurrent laryngeal nerve and hooking around the right subclavian artery. The right vagus then passes through the anterior to the right subclavian artery, running through the posterior to the superior vena cava, descends posterior to the right main bronchus, and contributes to the complexity of the cardiac, pulmonary, and esophageal plexuses. Forming the posterior vagal trunk at the lower part of the esophagus and it enters the diaphragm through the esophageal hiatus.

The left vagus nerve goes into the thorax between the left common carotid artery and left subclavian artery and descends on the aortic arch, which gives rise to the left recurrent laryngeal nerve, hooking around the aortic arch to the left of the ligamentum arteriosum, which then travels upwards in between the esophagus and trachea. Some thoracic-cardiac branches then branch from the left vagus and further break up into the pulmonary plexus, continuing into the esophageal plexus, and then make an entrance into the abdomen as the anterior part of the vagal trunk in the esophageal hiatus of the diaphragm.

The branches include; Pharyngeal nerve, Superior laryngeal nerve, Inferior cervical cardiac branch, Recurrent laryngeal nerve, Thoracic-cardiac branches, Branches to the pulmonary plexus, Branches to the esophageal plexus, Anterior vagal trunk, Posterior vagal trunk, Hering-Breuer reflex in alveoli

The vagus nerves run parallel between the common carotid artery and the internal jugular vein inside the carotid sheath.

Note; Plexus is a network of an interwoven mass of nerves, blood vessels, or lymphatic vessels.

Nuclei

The vagus nerve includes structurally long, thin fibers called "axons," which originate from the following four nuclei of the medulla:

1. The dorsal nucleus of the vagus nerve – this sends parasympathetic information to the internal organs that lay across the thoracic and abdominal cavity of the body, especially the gut.

2. The nucleus ambiguous – This gives rise to the brachial efferent motor fibers of the vagus nerve and preganglionic parasympathetic neurons that innervate the heart.

3. The solitary nucleus – which receives afferent taste information and primary afferents from visceral organs.

4. The spinal trigeminal nucleus – which receives sensory information about deep/crude touch, pain, and temperature of the

outer ear, the dura of the posterior cranial fossa, and the mucosa of the larynx.

Development

The motor functional part of the vagus nerve is gotten from the basal plate of the embryonic medulla oblongata, while the sensory functional part of the vagus nerve is derived from the cranial neural crest.

Functions of the Vagus Nerve

The vagus nerve is a very diverse nerve, and these are some of its functions:

1. It serves as a tool for the communication between the guts and the brain: The vagus nerve stands as a messenger between the gut and the brain. It conveys information from the gut about how the body is feeling to the brain for processing via electric impulses known as "action potentials."

2. It helps in reducing heart rate and blood pressure: The vagus nerve helps in lowering the heart rate due to its connection to the heart.

The vagus nerve has a close relationship with the heart. It is in charge of controlling the heart rate via electrical impulses to specialized cardiac muscle tissue known as the heart's natural pacemaker, which is in the right atrium, where "acetylcholine" is released to slow down the pulse.

3. It helps in fear management: The vagus nerve sends to the brain information from the gut, linked to stress, anxiety, and fear management. This helps a person recover from a scary or stressful

situation when faced or triggered by helping the person maintain calmness.

Best explained by saying that the vagus nerve initiates your body to relax.

When the sympathetic nervous system pours the stress hormone, cortisol, and adrenaline into your body, in the "fight or flight" responses. It is the vagus nerve that releases acetylcholine into the body, telling the body to relax. The tendrils of the vagus nerves extend to many organs and act like fiber-optic cables that send instructions to release enzymes and proteins like prolactin, vasopressin, and oxytocin, which calm you down. Vagus nerve response varies from individual to individual; for example, people with a weaker vagus response find it difficult to recover from injury, stress, or illness, while people with a much stronger vagus response may find it less difficult to recover rapidly.

4. Balancing of the nervous system: The nervous system is made up of two areas; first, the sympathetic area, which is responsible for the increment of alertness, energy, blood pressure, heart rate, and breathing and second, the parasympathetic in which the vagus nerve is heavily involved in, which helps in the decrement of the heart rate blood pressure, and alertness and it also helps with calmness, relaxation, and digestion. Therefore, the vagus nerve aids defecation, urination, and sexual arousals. Thereby helping to maintain a balance in the nervous system.

Mind you, even though it helps maintain balance in the nervous system, overstimulation of the vagus nerve can cause loss of consciousness

5. It helps in strengthening memory retainment: When the vagus nerve is stimulated, it releases into the amygdala the neurotransmitter norepinephrine, which helps strengthen memories. This, according to research and study, suggests a promising future treatment of conditions like Alzheimer's disease.

6. The vagus nerve prevents and decreases inflammation: The vagus nerve sends anti-inflammatory signals to other parts of the body. Inflammation is a physical condition that is sustained during or after injury or illness, and it is normal to have a certain amount of it, but too much inflammation is linked to many serious diseases and conditions, ranging from sepsis to the autoimmune condition rheumatoid arthritis. The vagus nerve gets a signal at the slightest detection of inflammation through its operation with a vast network of fibers stationed all around the body's organs.

In detecting the incipient inflammation —the presence of a substance called tumor necrosis factor (TNF)— alerts the brain and sends out anti-inflammatory neurotransmitters that regulate the body's immune response.

7. The vagus nerves help in the breathing process: The neurotransmitter acetylcholine, which the vagus nerve sends as a signal, informs your lungs to breathe, literally. To stimulate your vagus nerve, you can do that by yoga, meditation, abdominal breathing, or holding your breath for four to eight counts.

In summary, the vagus nerve, as described before, is a vast network of nerves that has a pathway to almost all the body's organs. Due to the connection and the active transmission of information from the brain to the organs or from the organs to the brain aids in the other functions as well; gag reflex, satiation after eating, vomiting, and fainting.

Effects of The Vagus Nerve

The vagus nerves have emotional effects on the body as well as physical effects.

1. The overstimulation of the vagus nerve in response to emotional stress can cause the overcompensation of the parasympathetic nervous system function to a strong sympathetic nervous system response linking with stress, which causes "vasovagal syncope." This causes the immediate drop of the blood pressure and heart rate and can cause uneasiness or trembling. During extreme vasovagal syncope, there are restrictions of blood flow to the brain, which leads to a shortage of blood supply to the brain, and one loses consciousness in the process. Although, most times, to make the symptoms subside, one has to sit or lie down for the necessary amount of time. Vasovagal syncope affects young children and women more than men.

2. It can also lead to temporary loss of bladder control under moments of extreme fear. That explains why when a person is faced with extreme situations that cause the person to fear, the person may urinate on himself/herself.

Research has proven that women having had complete spinal cord injury can still have orgasms through the vagus nerve, which can go from the uterus and cervix to the brain.

Vagus Nerve Stimulation (VNS)

The results obtained from the rigorous research and study made on the vagus nerve and its functions have birthed vagus nerve stimulation tested through clinical trials holds promises of a future of treatment and cure of serious, incurable disease.

Vagus Nerve Stimulation (VNS) is a medical procedure whereby the vagus nerve is stimulated either manually or by electrical pulses.

This has been used to try and treat a variety of conditions such as epilepsy, depression, rheumatoid arthritis, etc.

According to research, the effectiveness of Vagus Nerve Stimulation (VNS) has consequently been approved to be used in the treatment of epilepsy and mental illness.

Vagus Nerve Stimulation Implantation

This medical procedure, performed by a neurosurgeon, usually takes about 45-90 minutes with the patient most commonly under general anesthesia. Like with all surgeries, the patient stands a risk of infection, including inflammation or pain at the incision site, damage to nearby nerves, and constriction of nerves.

The medical procedure requires two small incisions for the implantation of the nerves. The first incision is made on the upper left side of the chest where the pulse generator is implanted, while the second one is made on the left side of the lower neck along a crease of the skin, where the thin, flexible wires (known as lead) that links the vague nerve to the pulse generator can be put in.

This device is a piece of metal that is flat and round and measures about 10-13 mm thick and 4 centimeters (an inch and a half) across.

This figure is dependent on the model because new models are much smaller.

The device contains a battery, which is made to last from one to 15 years, and when the battery is low, the device is replaced with a less invasive medical procedure which, this time, requires only the opening chest wall incision.

The device is usually activated after implantation, most commonly two to four weeks after implantation, although in some cases, it may be activated right in the operating room at the time of implantation. The device is usually programmed by the treating neurologist in his or her office with a small hand-held computer, programming wand, and programming software. During the programming, the strength and duration of the electrical impulses are programmed, although the quantity of stimulation varies according to the case but is usually initiated at a low level and gradually increased to a suitable level for the patient. The device works continuously and is programmed to switch on and shut off for specific programmed periods— for example, 25 seconds on and 6 minutes off.

The patients are provided with a Magnet Bracelet (handheld magnet) to control the device at home, in the workplace, or anywhere which must be activated and programmed by the treating neurologist to magnet mode. This works by delivering extra stimulation despise the programmed treatment schedule whenever the magnet is swept over the pulse generator site. To turn the device off, the magnet is held over the pulse generator while the magnet is in position while removing it will continue the stimulation cycle. All these maneuvers performed with the magnet can be done by the patient, family members, friends, or caregivers. Literally, it works like a remote control.

The side effects, most commonly related to stimulation, usually improve over time. These may include any of the following:

Hoarseness in the voice, coughing, tickling of the throat, and shortness of breath are the most common but are usually temporary.

This procedure can be used to treat the following:

1. Epilepsy

Epilepsy is a common condition that affects both ain abnormally and causes frequent unpredicted seizures.

Seizures are unpredictable bursts of electrical activity in the brain that affects how it works temporarily. They are characterized by a wide range of symptoms.

Epilepsy has no definite age at which it can occur, but usually, it starts either in childhood or in people over 60. It's most times lifelong but can get gradually better over time.

The treatment of epilepsy involves a small electrical device that is similar to a pacemaker. Under general anesthesia, the device (which has a thin wire called lead connecting it to the vagus nerve) is placed on the person's chest, which helps to send at regular intervals electrical impulses throughout the day to the brain via the vagus nerve.

Vagus Nerve Stimulation is proven to be effective, although it is faced with side effects:

1. Sore throat

2. Nausea/ Stomach Discomfort

3. Difficulty in swallowing

4. Shortness of breath

5. Change in voice by making it hoarse

6. Slow heart rate.

It is advised to report to your doctor if any of these symptoms start or persist as they may be ways to reduce or stop them.

2. Mental illness

Vagus Nerve Stimulation is used to treat drug-resistant cases of clinical depression, and it is found to help in the treatment in the following:

1. Alzheimer's disease: Since the vagus nerve helps one to make memories. This stimulation of the vagus nerve can release into the amygdala, neurotransmitter norepinephrine which strengthens memories. Thus this holds a promising future of treatment and cure of Alzheimer's disease.

2. Anxiety disorders: The vagus nerve helps in stress, anxiety, and fear management. Therefore, Vagus Nerve Stimulation can help in the treatment of anxiety disorders.

3. Rapid cycling bipolar disorder: This is a pattern of frequent, unique episodes in bipolar disorder. In "rapid cycling," a person with bipolar disorder experiences four or more distinct episodes of mania or depression in one year. It can unpredictably occur at any point and can come and go over many years depending on how well the disorder is being treated; it is not necessarily "permanent." The vagus nerve

has been proven to help in improving one's mood. Therefore, the therapy of stimulating the vagus nerve can help in the treatment of this disorder.

3. Inflammation

Inflammation usually occurs as a reaction to injury or infection. It is a localized physical condition in which part of the body becomes swollen, reddened, and often painful. Since it is known that the vagus nerve helps in decreasing inflammation when the vagus nerve sends an anti-inflammatory signal to the part or parts of the body that needs it. It is believed that Vagus Nerve Stimulation can be used in the treatment of inflammation.

Further research and consideration suggest that since the vagus nerve have pathways to almost all organs of the body, that it holds a promising future in the treatment of the following:

1. Inflammation from Crohn's disease, Parkinson's disease, diabetes mellitus, and rheumatoid arthritis.

2. Intractable hiccups

3. Abnormal heart rhythm and heart failure.

Although we were once saying the same thing for rheumatoid arthritis, now vagus nerve stimulation can be used in the treatment of rheumatoid arthritis, which helps reduce the symptoms to a significant level with no serious adverse side effects. Thus, it is believed that this procedure will be used, in the nearest future, to treat some serious, incurable diseases.

NOTES

Chapter 3:
Polyvagal Theory and Post Traumatic Stress Disorder (PTSD)

I t is clear that unpredictable PTSD has a solid neurological and physiological viewpoint to it. A comprehension of polyvagal theory gives a way to comprehend and enhance the terrible and regularly alarming substantial side effects that people living with complex PTSD endure. With a comprehension of the polyvagal theory set up, it turns into a matter of moral need to apply it to the manifestations and enduring of the individuals who have persevered through ceaseless maltreatment. Frequently during psychotherapy, people may end up encountering flashbacks and re-traumatization and be pitched into the conditions of hyperarousal or separation. This exposition contends that it is morally questionable to put patients through such terrible encounters without giving methods to enhance such terrifying manifestations. Patients are "urged to discuss the most agonizing occasions of their lives without helping them to adjust their excitement. That is clearly retraumatizing. Requesting that individuals remember the most loathsome experiences of their lives without showing them how to have a sense of security and quiet is risky to individuals' wellbeing; it is so off-base" (van der Kolk and Najavits, 2013, p. 521)

Information on the neurophysiological premise of complex PTSD symptomology is the basic way to furnish sufferers with a way to comprehend and adapt to the disrupting indications of injury. An examination into the social commitment framework's job in chemical imbalance (Bal et al., 2010), passionate guideline in marginal character issue (Austin, Riniolo, and Porges, 2007), and dissociative experience (Hart, 2013) recommend that that polyvagal theory can be applied very adequately to numerous clutters and ties numerous appearances of sick mental wellbeing together under a solitary recommended neurophysiological instrument. The polyvagal theory "has given one of a kind bits of knowledge into the job of feeling dysregulation in psychopathology, and into the advancement of unusual examples of autonomic sensory system working in various clinical disorders that before were viewed as disconnected" (Beauchaine, Gatzke-Kopp, and Mead, 2005, p. 181)

Further to its job in psychopathology, the polyvagal theory is a hopeful and positive way to deal with amplifying happiness for the most part in the human populace by applying procedures to down direct the crude, dread, and nervousness prompting old vagal reaction and advance the more current mammalian, social commitment frameworks that energize security and development in ideal social and network settings (Porges W. S., 2015). Information on polyvagal theory can be abused in two different ways: the logical power of the theory concerning the physical symptomology of complex PTSD in this way normalizing it and giving away to change psychological reaction to improve things and also, by taking care of mediations that diminishing the force of disagreeable physical side effects and advance a feeling of control by means of enactment of the characteristic quieting impact accessible from the parasympathetic sensory system.

NOTES

Chapter 4:
Trauma Recovery

M ost people who have suffered significant emotional trauma (e.g., the newly bereaved, citizens in war-torn countries, those who have been abused or sexually molested) or physical injury (e.g., extreme abuse, crippling disability) are emerging from their misfortune totally or almost fully. Some, though, do not do as well and, for an extended period, manage to relive the same horrific experiences of debilitating terror, depression, and panic. Their bad experiences have traumatized these latter groups of people.

In the book "Waking the Tiger: Healing Trauma," Levine and Frederick (1997) said it was the result of bottled-up somatosensory symptoms following trauma. "During a traumatic experience, there are three main ways people respond," Levine and Frederick (1997) said. They can fight (confront the situation), flee (get away from the situation), or freeze (be completely overwhelmed to the point of immobility by the predicament). Victims applying fighting or fleeing solutions to a traumatic experience are better at dealing with trauma than people freezing in response to shock (Levine & Frederick, 1997). This condition of suspended animation and paralysis occurs involuntarily and unconsciously. The patient has no means to go through all the usual responses correlated to traumatic events during this frozen condition (Levine & Frederick, 1997). The trapped emotions wreak havoc on the traumatized individual because the victim does not adequately release them. Therefore, the trauma solution is to guide the victim along a path (Experiential Sensation-FELT SENSE) that allows them to perceive and release those emotions that are trapped (Levine & Frederick, 1997). The therapeutic method is acquired from researching how pets rebound from traumatic experiences (Levine & Frederick 1997). Confronting trauma, Levine and Frederick (1997) said, should be mostly at an emotional, limbic level of the brain, not just at a rational, executive level of the brain.

The polyvagal theory, which suggests that trauma has a somatic experiential component, also supports Levine and Frederick's trauma theory in some ways. When, as the polyvagal hypothesis and the theory of Levine and Frederick (1997) suggest, trauma has strong emotional origins, features of partnership frameworks such as the DIR system can be implemented to resolve trauma. After determining the functional, emotional development capacity level of the victim, a DIR practitioner may begin to appeal, build and reinforce discovered areas of weaknesses, allowing the victim to escape from the shackling phenomena of a past traumatic event. Calming the traumatized individual is a tool for regulating traumatized individuals in the DIR toolbox. A calm mind creates an opportunity for further emotional regulation and understanding of deep-rooted feelings, all of which are needed for trauma victims to get out of the shackles of the past and begin to achieve new functional capacity heights.

Other relevant trauma theories include the NARM model, which, focused on the mind, suggests that trauma is associated with maladaptation in the history of the victim's attachment. The PTSD model suggests that trauma victims adopt approaches that have evolved and have been effective in the past for their current problems.

Throughout my view, while attachment and trauma seem like opposite ends of the same psychological spectrum, it is clear that while attachment is mostly optimistic, except in severe attachment/dependence situations, trauma is almost always destructive, at least until the person recovers. Trauma treatment requires a dedicated practitioner willing to learn from their victims and understand their challenges to develop a suitable management strategy.

Recognizing the signs and symptoms of injury, allowing prompt appointments to a trauma therapist, and incorporating several of the modalities mentioned above will likely yield the best outcome for treating distressed children and adults.

Why is the polyvagal theory very important?

For therapists and pop-psychology enthusiasts alike, understanding polyvagal theory can help with:

- Understanding trauma and PTSD

- Understanding Attack and withdrawal in relationships

- Understanding how extreme stress leads to dissociation or shutdown

- Understanding how to read body language

The truth is that emotions are responses (internal or external) to a stimulus. We sometimes happen out of our awareness, particularly if we are out of contact with our internal emotional life or incongruent with it.

To our bodies, our dominant desire to remain alive is more important than even our ability to think about staying alive. This is where the theory of polyvagism comes into play.

The nervous system always runs in the background, controlling our body functions to allow us to think about other things — like what ice cream we'd like to order or how to get that A in medical school. The entire nervous system works in tandem with the brain and, even if we don't want it, can take over our emotional experience.

A story about a gazelle

Animals are a great example of how we deal with stress because they react primarily without consciousness. They're doing what we'd do if we weren't tamed so well.

You've seen a lioness chase a gazelle if you've ever watched a National Geographic Africa special. A group of gazelles grazes, and suddenly one looks up, hyper-conscious of what's happening around him. The entire group is listening and paying attention.

The lioness ends her pursuit after a moment. She's singled out the gazelle, runs as fast as possible (sympathetic nervous system) until he's caught. He immediately goes stiff (parasympathetic nervous system) when he is captured.

The lioness drags the gazelle back to her cubs, where they start playing with her before heading in for slaughter. If the lioness gets distracted and the gazelle sees a moment of opportunity, he gets up and sprints off again, looking like he came back to life suddenly (back to the sympathetic response of the nervous system).

When the gazelle was captured, his reaction to the shutdown came in with fangs around his neck— he froze. The fight or flight came in when he saw the opportunity to run, so he did.

The polyvagal theory encompasses the three states— connection, difficulty, or run or shutdown.

Here's how it works:

Connection mode or... Rest and relaxation... Or myelinated vagus nerve: Myelinated vagus nerve of the parasympathetic nervous system flowing from the nucleus unclear reaction In non-stressful situations, if we are emotionally healthy, our bodies remain in a state of social involvement or a relaxed, natural, non-freaked-out mood.

I like to call it "connection." By connection, I mean we can interact with another human being "connected." We stroll outside, without doubt, loving our day, dining with friends and family, and feeling natural regarding our body and emotions.

It is also called the ventral vagal reaction, as this is the part of the brain triggered during the process of communication. It's like a normal life green light.

How do you see and feel this?

- We have a healthy immune system.
- We feel normal happiness, open-mindedness, peace, and life curiosity.
- We sleep well and eat normally.
- Our expression is flexible and articulate.

- We have an emotional relationship with others.

- We understand and listen to others more easily.

- We feel calm and rooted in our skin.

Freeze, flight, fight, or puff up... Or the sympathetic response of the nervous system: The sympathetic nervous system is our immediate response to stress, affecting almost every organ in the body.

The sympathetic nervous system causes the state we have all heard of "fight or flight." It gives us the signs to keep us alive.

How is this going to happen? How do you see and feel this?

- To search the atmosphere for real danger, we detect risk and freeze.

- We produce adrenaline, epinephrine, and norepinephrine to help us achieve what we need— get away from our opponent or battle it.

- We're sweating and feeling more mobilized.

- We're feeling anxious, scared, or angry.

- The metabolism slows down as the body is rushed for oxygen.

- Our blood vessels surround the intestines and dilate to the muscles required for running or battle.

- Our muscles may feel rigid, strong, tight, vibrating, doleful, shaking, and heavy.

- Maybe our hands are clammy.

- Our stomach can be knotted painfully.

- Our gestures can be seen as guarding our vital organs with our fists clenched or puffing up to look bigger or stronger.

Some people who have both traumas of attachment and subsequent trauma may experience chronic suicidality and episodes of dissociation that last days to months. Research shows that solutions for the long term include:

Dialectical behavioral treatment

Mentalization-based therapy

Transition oriented counseling where trauma affects the nervous system

If we experience emotional or physical danger, we do the same thing as that gazelle. We alternate between peaceful grazing (parasympathetic mode of connection), fighting or flight (sympathetic system of fighting and flight), or shutdown (parasympathetic mode of shutdown).

The reaction is everything when it comes to trying to understand the situation. Perhaps when they leaped out to scare us, somebody was just playing a game, but we fainted. Whatever the cause, whether or not the accident was malicious, our body switched in shutdown mode; we reported it as an injury. Our body moved to shutdown mode.

Or perhaps the injury incident was life-threatening, and our nervous system reacted to the stimulus accordingly.

No matter what the trigger is, our subconscious concluded that what was going on was life-threatening enough to force our body to run or freeze.

If someone has been through such a traumatic event that their body tips into shutdown mode, any incident that reminds the person of that life-threatening occurrence may again cause them to isolate or break down.

People can even live for days or months at a time in a state of disconnection or shutdown.

At intense, sudden noises like explosions or thunderstorms, vets sometimes feel that. A woman who has been raped may switch to hyper-vigilant or dissociated response quickly if she feels someone is following her. Someone who has been violated may go into shock when even another person begins to yell.

The problem occurs when the initial trauma has not been handled in such a manner as to address the original trauma.

That's what PTSD (post-traumatic stress disorder) is — the overreaction of our body to a small response, either stuck or shut down in combat and flight.

People who experience injury and the reaction to shutdown usually feel guilty for their inability to act while their body has not changed. Often they wish they had fought more in those moments.

Vietnam veterans could believe their comrades who died around them, frozen with terror, lost. Victims of rape may believe that they may have not resisted their attacker because they have frozen.

Victims of abuse can believe that they are not trying to escape from their attacker and are either powerless or failing.

A lot of "pressure" practice, which teaches people to stay in battle and flight mode, aims to keep people out of dissociation in actual life or death situations. Unfortunately, in contrast to elite sports teams or Special Forces, such activities are not popular. The right amount of stress, with good recovery, can lead to higher levels of adaptation of our nervous systems.

Coming out of shutdown mode

So how do we get back out of shutdown mode?

The dorsal vagal system's opposite is the system of social engagement.

So, in short, what fixes shutdown mode is to bring somebody into a healthy social commitment or a proper attachment.

Looking into the nuts and bolts of how this happens in our bodies will help us understand why when the body is in battle, flight, or shut down mode, we feel the way we do physically.

We will learn how to change states as we realize what the body reacts the way it does, like a series of instructions and some basic brain science. We should start moving out of the system of fight or flight, out of the style of withdrawal, and back into the state of social engagement.

Whether we are only developing a bond with a young, nervous client or helping them cope with their most traumatic memories as counselors, it is important to know how to handle the polyvagal systems.

It may also be useful because, in some of these signs, you have just found yourself. Such as, "When I'm with my family, even as an adult when they start fighting, I feel light-headed and detached." If you've experienced some of these issues for yourself, perhaps by counseling and even knowing how it functions, you will get yourself out of a disconnected condition.

Studies show that some parts of the brain, including verbal centers and brain reasoning centers, shut down during the recall of traumatic events (Van Der Kolk, 2006).

That's why it's important to conduct therapy in a safe, healthy way, in a safe, healthy environment, or to come out of shutdown mode. That is why it is imperative to have a positive attachment. Or you run the risk of the person getting retraumatized.

Because I'm a psychiatrist, I'll write this to show how to help a patient switch off shutdown mode.

These tips, however, still apply to those who only understand how the shutdown mode works. And it can even encourage those who feel shut down and continue trying to get back to a balanced style of social engagement.

Have a relationship of trust. Due to the potential of re-traumatization, don't even discuss intensively traumatic events— especially those where you believe disconnect mode has set in until the therapeutic partnership feels deeply linked.

As a psychologist, it's important to allow the client to express things that they couldn't communicate with others— shameful thoughts, rage, sexual response, anything that seems scared to share with others.

Find a quiet center of your own. You're throwing them a lifeline if you can empathize with their distress, stay with them in the moment and help them feel connected during their shutdown. You help them get out of the freeze through social engagement.

Combating the desire to dissociate is essential, no matter how gruesome the topic is. As psychologists, because of the mirror neuron reaction, we might dissociate — to mimic the brain of our client, and because it's easy to imagine it occurring to us when experiencing traumatic pain.

The human experience is so powerful that it rewrites that event in our brain when we re-engage the trauma with someone else to support us, adding to the feeling of being supported in the memory of the trauma. We are creating new neural pathways around the trauma, and we can change the response of our body to it.

Let that guide the client. Don't go looking for a witch. Step into the topic if the client brings it up. But, by asking leading questions and trying to get them to confess, it is harmful to prompt the patient into something that is not there. Do not allow your own experience to lead you to imagine that they have experienced something as well.

Standardize your answers. The whole principle of polyvagism would allow one to say "thank you!" To the organs of us. Even if that process is at times overactive — unwarranted fear or anxiety — which our body watches over us, trying to keep us safe.

The skin is the same as the gazelle, either running away or limping. And in the first instance, gazelles have no concept of what feelings are.

Now that the patient understands that their emotional response has been adaptive, primal, and suitable, we can get rid of the shame caused by their non-reaction.

Support them to understand their frustration. Anger is an incredibly adaptive emotion, and we don't allow ourselves to have it. We think it's bad for anger. Yet rage also tells us where we breached our healthy boundaries.

Anger fills us with the power to conquer the barrier. They would make the person understand that they had to resolve the emotional energy, but at the time they wanted to, the strength could not be reflected.

If we can get a person to recognize their frustration in a meeting, they will see that the traumatic event was not completely unresponsive. If we can help them feel even the tiniest twitch of a micro-expression of anger on their face— the subtle lowering of the internal eyebrows— we will reassure them that in that moment, their body did not completely deceive them.

They should reconcile their desires with their bodies and thoughts. This helps develop a state of congruence— where their inner feelings align specific thoughts to their external displays.

Furthermore, as a dissociative memory is explored, feeling anger and shame reduction allows the memory to change fundamentally.

Introduce the motion of the skin. Since shutdown allows us to stop, it is a great way to reactivate body movements when thinking about the pain and reconnect the body and mind to get them out of shutdown.

One of my clients, for example, was in an incident. When the EMS arrived, she was secured to a gurney for charging into an ambulance's rear. More than the actual accident, she felt pain being stuck on that gurney. She was afraid that she would injure her neck during the whole ride to the hospital, and all the stress about a neck injury led her to be paralyzed in terror.

In the therapy session, even talking about the trauma, her body was stiff, frozen, and dissociated.

I asked her, "During that time, how would you want to move?"She said she wanted to be able to lift her legs. I asked her to move her hands deliberately, attentively, the way she wanted to.

It is necessary to deliberately and gradually do the motion, concentrating on the movement's sensation. That patient felt an enormous energy release. She was able to tell the experience as a story in the subsequent treatments, rather than dissociating.

Making the client push— slow hitting, jumping, spinning, and gradually moving in place— flips the individual from shutdown into battle or flight mode, with the aim being to switch into contact or social engagement mode.

Exercises in body movement can fundamentally change the memory in conjunction with talking to a therapist.

Practice reinforcement. In relationships where one person feels they cannot connect well with the other person, an emotional breakdown can occur.

This behavior was defined as stonewalling by one psychologist, John Gottman. Practicing assertiveness may make the client feel more in control of their psychological situation and feel safe to move into habits of healthy relationships.

Breathing practice, mindfulness, and meditation all play a role in becoming more integrated with your body here and now.

Practice strength training and become a Judo Master. It can be important and educate yourself on how to protect yourself better in the future and also, over time, reset the anxiety cycle.

NOTES

Chapter 5:
The Healing Power of Vagal Tone

T he Polyvagal Theory has effectively linked the physical and emotional. Physical actions can regulate emotional conditions, emotional activities can cause physical responses. For example, deep, forceful, diaphragmatic breathing can initiate a state of deep calm, while emotional reactions can lead to stress, triggering elevated heart rate and respiratory rates and a range of other visceral organ reactions, such as stopping digestion as a form of energy conservation. Given the role of the vagus nerve in mediating both physical and emotional reactions, it is no surprise that the vagus nerve can be engaged to better manage our emotional sense of wellbeing and help alleviate physical problems.

As we have seen, under normal conditions, the calming parasympathetic nervous system is dominant, keeping the body in a state of homeostasis. In this context, a vagal tone is an assessment of the body's readiness to perform certain key functions effectively. An ideal vagal tone maintains a baseline from inputs via the vagus nerve received from the parasympathetic nervous system. Among the most important vagal tone functions is controlling heart rate to keep it from beating too quickly. Vagal activity is key to controlling breathing rate, managing the rate of peristaltic contractions during digestion, and further affecting the sensitivities and inflammation of the digestive tract and functioning of the liver. Vagal tone is also a measurement of emotional stability, as emotions form their basis of normalcy when the dorsal vagal and ventral vagal responses are at homeostasis.

But this is not always the case, especially when emotional reactions ignite physiological responses.

Regulating Emotion

The parasympathetic nervous system follows two pathways. The better known, and far more dominant, is the ventral vagal pathway that controls most of the key organ functions. As noted above, it encourages social engagement and interaction to further secure and stabilize the individual. The more recently recognized but older pathway, the dorsal vagal, controls the emergency freeze response, which causes immobility, lightheadedness, speechlessness, fainting, and shock. While the ventral vagal parasympathetic response is mediated by the neocortex, the newly-discovered and most developed part of the brain, the dorsal vagal parasympathetic response is mediated or activated by the most primitive, reptilian part of the brain.

Malfunctioning of either of these vagal pathways can lead to emotional disturbances, but regulating the vagal tone can moderate them. Brain function, specifically emotional responses and reactions, is directly affected by signals carried by the vagus nerve. Studies have shown that behavioral measures of emotional expression, emotional disturbances, self-regulatory skills, and reactivity may be correlated with baseline cardiovascular levels of vagal tone, leading to the conclusion that cardiovascular vagal tone can indicate how well emotions are being regulated and managed. This perspective was not considered traditionally until the Polyvagal Theory opened this enlightened perspective and continues to encourage further experimentation.

The higher the level of vagal tone, the healthier the baseline condition of mind and body. Therefore, given the direct relationship between physical and emotional conditions, it follows that practicing the exercises to improve physical vagal tone will contribute to the improvement of emotional conditions, returning them to more normal baseline levels.

Emotional conditions that may be the consequence of low vagal tone include anxiety, depression, sensations of stress, fatigue not caused by excessive activity, and sleeplessness. Other, more long-lasting emotional conditions may include Post Traumatic Stress Disorder (PTSD) and Attention Deficit Hyperactivity Disorder (ADHD). While many of these emotional disorders may respond to professional counseling and prescribed medication, hard-to-treat cases may respond favorably to vagal toning activities.

Physical actions that can return the body's emotional and physical reactions to normal baseline levels include Yoga stretches and poses, various forms of meditation, oral exercises to stimulate the vagus nerve in proximity to the vocal cords, cold water to the face, auricular massaging of the ears and earlobes and sides of the neck to stimulate the vagus nerve as it passes through the ears and along the carotid arteries. Practicing mindfulness, or being in the moment is a variation on meditation with awareness of every environment stimulus.

The effectiveness of all of these exercises can be enhanced by managed diaphragmatic breathing with deep, deliberate, thoughtful inhales and exhales, which directly stimulate the vagus nerve. The effect is to slightly increase the heart rate on inhales and lower heart rate back to a healthy or homeostatic baseline on exhales.

When the vagal tone is high, physical and emotional states are normal. With low vagal tone, the consequence of not stimulating the vagus nerve can result in a wide range of emotional disorders and, additionally, can contribute to a sense of apathy, loneliness, isolation, and a host of other negative moods. These are all symptoms of the inability to engage socially and participate in social interaction. This may continue a self-perpetuating downward spiral, with the sense of isolation tending to discourage social interaction and with the disconnection from social engagements furthering the feelings of isolation. Low vagal tone can also cause cardiovascular disorders.

Cardiovascular Applications

The relationship between the vagus nerve and the heart has been extensively researched and verified, with further clarification emerging from the Polyvagal Theory.

To set the stage for understanding this relationship, let's begin with the physical side of the relationship.

The vagus nerve travels from the brainstem and connects with the heart muscle or myocardium on the upper right side of the heart, in a cluster of nerves called the sinus node, for short, or sinoatrial node. Here the vagus nerve acts like a natural pacemaker, regulating the heartbeat. During normal conditions, at times of homeostasis, when there is little or no activity or stress, signals arriving from the brain through the vagus nerve slow the heart rate to less than 100 beats per minute. It is subsequently slowed and regulated, sequentially, by the atrioventricular node, the bundle of His, the right and left bundle branches, and finally the Purkinje fibers at the bottom of the myocardium. Every second or so, the heart muscle contracts, blood is forced out of the ventricles toward the lungs from the right ventricle and into the aorta from the left ventricle.

Now, here is where the relationship between the heart and emotional reactions occur, but first, a quick background. The Polyvagal Theory has added clarity to our understanding of how the autonomic nervous system in primates evolved from the more primitive reptile nervous system. Changes evolved to accommodate the more complex primate nervous system, resulting in increasingly elaborate vagal pathways that control or regulate the heart. There was a transition from the exclusive dorsal vagus nucleus among reptiles to a more elaborate structure in mammals, called the nuclear ambiguous.

This included a connection between the heart and the face that enabled social interactions to influence the visceral or bodily functions and possible dysfunctions. In simple terms, this means that social activity and other emotionally regulated activities could play a role in maintaining control over the heart rate, while conversely, cardiovascular events can directly affect emotions.

Charles Darwin, the founder of evolutionary theory, recognized the bi-directional flow between the brain and the heart that is mediated by the vagus nerve. Darwin understood that facial expressions were a physical manifestation of emotions and correctly surmised that neural pathways were connecting the brain with the heart and other organs that would facilitate physiological responses to emotions. Darwin and those of his time were correct in their estimate, despite not yet knowing that the pneumogastric nerve, later renamed the

57

vagus nerve, had its own private network connection between the brain and the heart, apart from the connections of the action-oriented sympathetic nervous system. Capabilities to elevate and reduce heart rate coexist.

A simple but effective determination of vagal tone is a measurement of the heart rate during inhalation when it should increase slightly above baseline, and then measurement of the heart rate during exhalation, when the heart rate should return to baseline. The different rates of the two heart rates can be used to specify the precise vagal tone.

What does this mean to you?

During times of stress, your physical side may be in a state of elevated heart and respiratory rate, and you may be sweating, feeling a need to exert yourself and take action. In those situations when the cause of the sympathetic response is alleviated, and there is no need to run, or fight, or jump, you can cool things down, calm your body with thoughts of calm, peace, reassurance. Repeat to yourself that everything is okay, under control, and it's okay to relax.

NOTES

Chapter 6:
Autoimmune Responses and
Inflammation

A relationship has been established between the autonomic nervous system (ANS) and the body's inflammatory response. It has long been understood that the autoimmune system includes inflammation as part of its responses to infection since inflammation helps trigger many aspects of the body's defense, including the release of macrophages or white blood cells and killer T-cells that identify and annihilate invading microorganisms. But often, the autoimmune system can overreact and overwork, continuing inflammation to the point where it can become damaging.

Non-drug treatments to calm the autoimmune responses are being derived from Polyvagal Theory. One approach is rocking, that is, a rocking motion in a chair or on a cushion. This is believed to have a soothing effect overall and a stimulating effect on carotid baroreceptors. Recall that vagal tone can be increased by massaging the vagus nerve on both sides of the neck, where the vagus nerve runs past the carotid arteries. As a result of steady, continuous rocking several times a day for several days, blood pressure levels are lowered as the relaxation functions of the parasympathetic nervous system are engaged.

Another relaxant of the autoimmune response involves contractions of the pelvic floor in a manner similar to contractions of the diaphragm. But while the diaphragm controls the upper body functions of the lungs and respiratory system, the pelvic floor holds the lower body, including the bladder and colon. An exercise to contract and engage the pelvic floor involves sitting on an exercise ball and feeling the pelvic floor begin to relax and settle into the ball, then trying to tighten it, then releasing it, letting it settle again, and repeating the cycle.

Dr. Stephen Porges, the founder of Polyvagal Theory, also advocates standing on a half-exercise ball with a rounded bottom and flat top, with someone else holding your hand to steady and give reassurance. This not only facilitates the therapeutic benefits of the balancing effort but also introduces a social engagement function, which signals the calming parasympathetic nervous system to initiate the socially engaging and relaxing ventral vagal response.

Added to these targeted, specific exercises can be the group of actions that have been used for other situations where the fight or flight sympathetic nervous system has engaged and needs to be turned down, or whenever the dorsal vagal response creates immobility, lightheadedness, and more severe freeze symptoms. These include Yoga poses and stretches, meditation, vigorous cardiovascular exercises, massage of the neck and ears, cold facial therapy, and, importantly, diaphragmatic deep, conscious breathing.

Autoimmune reactions discussed here are moderate and are not at the level of being serious, chronic, or life-threatening. But in cases of more serious autoimmune disorders, there is no substitute for professional medical treatment. The critical first step is the correct diagnosis of the condition and identification of its cause.

Our contemporary ingestion of medications for numerous conditions, both real and imagined, can lead to bodily reactions, notably autoimmune overreactions. This may be exacerbated by taking herbal supplements, which can conflict with medications being taken, or that might initiate autoimmune disorders on their own:

Herbal supplements are lightly regulated by the Food and Drug Administration (FDA), and marketers may not be fully cognizant of potential side effects. Anyone taking prescription medications should check with their physician or pharmacist before mixing their medications with herbs.

NOTES

Chapter 7:
Clinical Applications of Polyvagal Theory

Facial Expressions, Asperger's Spectrum, and Autism

T he Polyvagal Theory addresses the treatment of autistic and other, less extremely affected Asperger's Spectrum children, with the presupposition that these children's social interaction capabilities are physically undamaged and may be awakened with the right type of stimulation. Given that many of these afflicted children are unable to control their social behaviors, or more precisely, unable or unwilling to activate and use their social behavior voluntarily, the Polyvagal Theory holds that there are ways to stimulate the vagus nerve in ways that can encourage the children to manifest the physical dimensions of social engagement.

The Polyvagal model assumes that for many Asperger's children with social communication deficits, including those at the extreme end who are diagnosed with autism, their social engagement systems are intact and are not missing or have irredeemably damaged components of their central nervous systems.

In recalling the earlier discussion of neuroception, this is a concept with the purpose of analyzing and interpreting certain environmental factors and then initiating either defensive reactions or stimulating the onset of the calming reaction. An example is the function of neural circuits that enable a child to smile and respond positively when they recognize someone familiar but to hesitate or flee from an unknown stranger. These reactions are common among all children and can be overcome by simple reassurances.

But in situations involving Autism and less extreme Asperger's Spectrum disorders, the goal is to find ways to arouse or initiate the positive responses to the familiar and suppress the escape or avoidance tendencies that are almost always functioning. The autistic and Asperger's children, according to Polyvagal Theory, are in a permanent state of fear-inducing unfamiliarity and need to be drawn out.

It has been found that autistic and Asperger's children may be engaged socially by the use of encouraging, reassuring facial expressions, altering neuroception. In test situations, it is found that the social inhibition of children with autism may be less of a physical disorder than a purely emotional reaction to stress. If this is correct, it may be theoretically possible to associate their symptoms with either low-level sympathetic defensive responses to stress and fear or possibly due to dorsal vagal freeze immobilization. The combination of facial expressions, especially wide, sincere smiling and eyes wide open, eye contact, and reassuring speaking, can begin to give autistic children a sense that they can trust someone and begin to socially interact with the person. This is consistent with other studies that have demonstrated that social engagement can contribute to the calming, relaxing parasympathetic response.

In contrast, however, new studies are finding that certain brain anomalies can inhibit facial recognition in autistic children and teenagers. In these instances, there is a physical barrier that increases autism symptoms and reduces the potential for facial expression therapy to be effective.

Vagus Nerve Dietary and Nutritional Influences

Among the newer discoveries that involve the vagus nerve, studies are drawing a vagal connection between what we eat and how the brain responds.

New research into obesity control and the role of various types of diets and foods has identified a unique and important role of the vagus nerve in transmitting data from the stomach to the brain. The vagus nerve connects to nerves in the stomach and sends that afferent data to inform the brain of the caloric value, or potential energy, of the stomach's contents. These data, in turn, causes the brain to either suppress appetite-stimulating hormones when calorie counts are high or to increase these hormones when the calorie content is low.

Controlled studies have been conducted among volunteers who agreed to hospital confinement so their exact consumption behavior can be accurately recorded. The usual method of having study participants record their eating experiences in a diary has been found to be highly inaccurate.

The researchers have discovered that the data forwarded to the brain by the vagus nerve can be distorted by over-processed foods and especially by artificial sweeteners. In the case of saccharine-type sugar substitutes, the part of the brain responsible for decision-making, the striatum, is misinformed, interpreting the afferent information to mean there is a specific energy potential available in the gut. When the expected energy is not available, the brain actually becomes confused and encourages more eating, leading to the ingestion of excessive calories.

In an environment of many, often conflicting, dietary recommendations and claims, each purporting to be ideal diets for health and weight control, these new findings strongly discourage diets overly based on over-processed foods and dietary consumption of artificial sweeteners. Natural, unprocessed, whole foods, long the standard of our evolutionary ancestors, remain the more responsible nutritional choice.

NOTES

Chapter 8:
Yoga Therapy And Polyvagal Theory

Yoga therapy is a recently developing, automatic correlative and integrative human service (CIH) practice. It is developing in its professionalization, acknowledgment, and use with a showed responsibility to setting practice principles, instructive and accreditation norms, and elevating exploration to help its viability for different populaces and conditions.

In any case, heterogeneity of training, poor detailing principles, and absence of an extensively acknowledged comprehension of the neurophysiological systems associated with yoga treatment restrain the organizing of testable speculations and clinical applications.

Currently proposed structures of yoga-themed practices center concerning the combination of base up neurophysiological and top-down neurocognitive components. What's more, it has been suggested that phenomenology and first individual moral request can give a focal point through which yoga treatment is seen as a procedure that contributes towards eudaimonic prosperity in the experience of torment, sickness, or incapacity. In this chapter, we expand on these systems and propose a model of yoga treatment that merges with Polyvagal Theory (PVT).

PVT joins the development of the autonomic sensory system to the rise of prosocial practices and states that the neural stages supporting social conduct are engaged with looking after wellbeing, development, and reclamation. This logical model, which associates neurophysiological examples of autonomic guidelines and articulation of enthusiastic and social conduct, is progressively used as a system for understanding human conduct, stress, and disease.

In particular, we portray how PVT can be conceptualized as a neurophysiological partner to the yogic ideal of the gunas or characteristics of nature. Like the neural stages portrayed in PVT, the gunas give the establishment from which conduct, passionate and physical traits rise. We depict how these two distinct yet closely resembling structures - one situated in neurophysiology and the other in an old intelligence convention - feature yoga treatment's advancement of physical, mental, and social prosperity for self-guideline and strength. This parallel between the neural foundation of PVT and the gunas of yoga is instrumental in making a translational structure for yoga treatment to line up with its philosophical establishments. Thusly, yoga treatment can work as a particular practice instead of fitting into an outside model for its usage in inquires about its clinical settings.

Mind-body treatments, including yoga treatment, are proposed to profit wellbeing and prosperity through reconciliation of top-down and base-up forms encouraging bidirectional correspondence between the cerebrum and body. Top-down procedures, for example, the guideline of consideration and setting of expectation, have been shown to diminish mental worry just as hypothalamic-pituitary pivot (HPA) and thoughtful sensory system movement (SNS), and thusly balance insusceptible capacity and irritation. Base-up forms, advanced by breathing procedures and development rehearsals, have been appeared to impact the musculoskeletal, cardiovascular and sensory system work and furthermore influence HPA and SNS movement with frequent changes in resistant capacity and passionate prosperity.

The top-down and base-up forms utilized at the top of the body treatment priorities list may control autonomic, neuroendocrine, enthusiastic, and conduct actuation and bolster a person's reaction to challenges. Self-guideline, a cognizant capacity to keep up the security of the framework by overseeing or modifying reactions to risk or misfortune, may diminish the side effects of differing conditions.

Versatility may give another advantage of mind-body treatments as it incorporates the capacity of a person to "ricochet back" and adjust in light of affliction as well as unpleasant conditions in an opportune manner to such an extent that psychophysiological assets are rationed. High strength is related to faster cardiovascular recuperation following abstract passionate encounters, less seen pressure, more noteworthy recuperation from ailment or injury, and better administration of dementia and incessant agony. Traded off versatility is connected to dysregulation of the autonomic sensory system through proportions of vagal guidelines (respiratory sinus arrhythmia). Yoga is related to both improvements in proportions of mental strength and improved vagal guidelines.

This article investigates the mix of top-down and base-up forms for self-guideline and versatility through Polyvagal Theory and yoga treatment. PVT will be portrayed in connection to contemporary understandings of interoception as the biobehavioral hypothesis of the "preliminary set," which will be characterized later. This will help spread out an incorporated framework to see which mind-body treatments encourage the development of physiological, enthusiastic, and social qualities for the advancement of self-guideline and strength.

We will look at the union of the neural stages, depicted in PVT, with the three Gunas, a fundamental idea of the yogic way of thinking that portrays the characteristics of material nature. Both PVT and yoga give structures to seeing how basic neural stages (PVT) and gunas (yoga) interface the development and availability between physiological, mental, and conduct characteristics. By influencing the neural stage, or guna transcendence, just as one's relationship to the ceaseless moving of these neural stages, or gunas, the individual learns aptitudes for self-guideline and strength. In addition, these structures share qualities that parallel each other where the neural stage mirrors the guna power, and the guna prevalence reflects the neural stage.

PVT, and other rising hypotheses, for example, neurovisceral combination, help explain associations between the frameworks of the body, the cerebrum, and the procedures of the mind offering expanded understanding into complex examples of incorporated top-down and base up forms that are natural to mind-body treatments. PVT portrays three particular neural stages in light of apparent hazard (i.e., wellbeing, peril, and life-risk) in the conditions that work in a phylogenetically decided chain of command, steadily with the Jacksonian guideline of disintegration. PVT acquaints the idea of neuroception with depicting the subliminal recognition of wellbeing or peril in nature through base up forms including vagal afferents, tangible info identified with outside difficulties, and endocrine components that recognize and assess ecological hazard before the cognizant elaboration by higher mind focuses.

The three polyvagal neural stages, as portrayed underneath, are connected to the practices of social correspondence, guarded procedure of activation, and protective immobilization:

1. The ventral vagal complex (VVC) gives the neural structures that intervene in the "social commitment framework." At the point when wellbeing is recognized in the interior and outside condition, the VVC gives a neural stage to help prosocial conduct and social association by connecting the neural guideline of instinctive states supporting homeostasis and reclamation to facial expressivity and the open and expressive areas of correspondence (e.g., prosodic vocalizations and upgraded capacity to tune in to voice). The engine segment of the VVC, which starts in the core ambiguous (NA), manages and organizes the muscles of the face and head with the bronchi and heart. These associations help prepare the individual towards human association and commitment in prosocial connections and give increasingly adaptable and versatile reactions to ecological difficulties, including social communications

2. The SNS is often connected with battle/flight practices. Battle/flight practices require initiation of the SNS and are the underlying and essential guard procedures enlisted by warm-blooded creatures. This safeguard technique requires expanded metabolic yield to help activation practices. Inside PVT, the enlistment of SNS on guard pursues the Jacksonian guideline of disintegration and mirrors the versatile responses of a phylogenetically

requested reaction progressively in which the VVC has neglected to alleviate risk. When the SNS circuit is selected, there are monstrous physiological changes remembering an expansion for muscle tone, shunting of blood from the fringe, restraint of gastrointestinal capacity, an enlargement of the bronchi, increments in pulse and respiratory rate, and the arrival of catecholamines.

This assembly of physiological assets makes way for reacting to genuine or accepted peril in the earth and towards the ultimate objectives of security and endurance. When the SNS turns into the predominant neural stage, the VVC impact might be repressed for activating assets for a quick activity. Though prosocial practices and social association are related to the VVC, the SNS is related to practices and feelings, for example, dread or outrage, that helps to prepare the earth for security or wellbeing.

3. The dorsal vagal complex (DVC) emerges from the dorsal core of the vagus (DNX) and gives the essential vagal engine filaments to organs situated beneath the stomach. This circuit is intended to adaptably react to massive peril or dread and is the crudest (i.e., developmentally most established) reaction to stretch. Initiation of the DVC in resistance brings about an uninvolved reaction portrayed by diminished muscle tone and an emotional decrease of heart yield to save metabolic assets and modification in gut and bladder work by means of reflexive poop and pee to lessen metabolic requests required by processing.

PVT states that through these neural stages: specific physiological states, mental traits, and social procedures are associated, develop, and are made open to the person. The physiological state built up by these neural stages in light of risk or security (as decided through the coordinated procedures of neuroception) takes into consideration or limits the scope of passionate and social attributes that are open to the person

A center part of PVT is that examples of physiological state, feeling, and conduct are specific to each neural stage (for a point-by-point audit of the neurophysiological, neuroanatomical, and developmental natural bases of PVT. For instance, the neural foundation of the VVC is proposed to associate instinctive homeostasis with passionate qualities and prosocial practices that are contradictory to the neurophysiological states, enthusiastic attributes, or social practices that show in the neural foundation of protective procedures found in SNS or DVC initiation. When the VVC is predominant, the vagal brake is executed, and prosocial practices and enthusiastic states, for example, association and love, can possibly develop.

When the SNS is the essential guarded system, the NA kills the inhibitory activity of the ventral vagal pathway to the heart to empower thoughtful enactment, and in turn, social and passionate procedures of assembly are bolstered. On the off chance, the DVC idleness reaction is the cautious system, the dorsal engine core is initiated as a defensive component from agony or potential demise, which means dynamic reaction methodologies are not accessible.

It is imperative to note that the VVC has different qualities that empower mixed states with the SNS (e.g., play) or with the DVC (e.g., closeness). Be that as it may, in these instances of mixed states, the VVC remains effectively available and practically contains the subordinate circuits. When the VVC is pulled back, it advances the availability of the SNS as a guard battle/flight framework. Also, the SNS practically restrains access to the DVC immobilization shutdown reaction. In this way, the significant shutdown response that may prompt demise becomes neurophysiologically available just when the SNS is reflexively repressed.

Vagal Activity, Interception, Regulation, and Resilience

Vagal movement, via ventral vagal pathways, is recommended to be an intelligent guideline for the versatility of the framework where high heart vagal tone is associated with increasingly versatile top-down and base-up procedures; for example, consideration guidelines, full of feeling preparation and adaptability of physiological frameworks to adjust and react to the earth. Vagal control has additionally been shown to relate with differential actuation in mind locales that manage reactions to risk evaluation, interoception, feeling guidelines, and the advancement of more noteworthy adaptability in light of challenge. On the other hand, the low vagal guideline has been related with maladaptive base up and top-down handling bringing about poor self-guideline, less social adaptability, discouragement, conclusive uneasiness issues, and antagonistic wellbeing results remembering expanded mortality for conditions, for example, lupus, rheumatoid joint pain, and injury.

Self-guideline is proposed to be subject to the precision with which we decipher and react to interoceptive data, with more prominent exactness prompting upgraded versatility and self-guideline. Thusly, interoception is viewed as significant in torment, habit, enthusiastic guideline, and solid, versatile practices, including social commitment. Furthermore, interoception has been proposed as key to versatility as the precise preparation of interior substantial states advancing a brisk rebuilding of homeostatic parity.

It has been suggested that mind-body treatments are a successful device for the guideline of vagal capacity, with results encouraging towards of versatile capacities including the alleviation of unfavorable impacts related to social difficulty, the decrease of allostatic load, and the assistance of self-administrative abilities and strength of the ANS crosswise over different patient populaces and conditions.

Polyvagal Theory & Mind-Body Therapies for Regulation & Resilience

Mind-body treatments underscore the development of physical mindfulness, including both interoception and proprioception, joined with the care-based characteristics of non-judgment, non-reactivity, interest, or acknowledgment so as to take part in a procedure of re-evaluation of improvements. While being urged to develop familiarity with BME wonders and boosts, the individual is bolstered in a procedure of re-elucidation or re-direction to such improvements so understanding may happen and flexibility, guideline, and versatility might be cultivated.

This ability to change the relationship and response to BME wonders is believed to be fundamental for self-guideline and prosperity. It has been indicated that patients using mind-body treatments for recuperating revealed both a move as far as they can tell and reaction to negative feelings and sensations similar to the improvement of self-administrative aptitudes in managing torment, enthusiastic guideline and re-examination of life circumstances.

PVT offers knowledge into how to figure out how to perceive and move the hidden neural foundation of any given psychophysiological state may legitimately influence physiology, feeling, and conduct, along these lines helping the individual develop versatile procedures for guideline and flexibility to profit physical, mental, and social wellbeing. As mind-body treatments influence the vagal pathways, they are proposed to shape methods for "working out" these neural stages to encourage self-guideline and strength of physiological capacity, feeling guideline, and prosocial practices.

Ideal neural guideline of the autonomic sensory system and the related endocrine and invulnerable frameworks is encouraged through a dynamic commitment of the VVC by using explicit developments or positions, breathing works on, reciting, or contemplation which influences both top-down and base-up forms.

Versatility is proposed to be cultivated by both downregulating cautious states and supporting greater adaptability and flexibility in relation to different wonders of the BME to advance physiological rebuilding just as positive mental and social states. The individual can figure out how to improve the actuation of the VVC with its homeostatic effect on the living being, similar to increment in the office to move all the way through other neural stages, for example, the SNS or DVC when genuine or seen pressure is experienced.

In total, personality body practices can show the person to make the VVC increasingly open, extend the limit of resilience to other neural stages, change the relationship and reaction to SNS and DVC neural stages that happen as common vacillations of the BME, and how to turn out to be progressively talented at moving all through these neural stages. Breathing moves inside yoga regularly encourage comparable moves in the autonomic state with focalized mental and wellbeing outcomes. These practices may likewise add to our capability to encounter association past social communications or systems and to a progressively all-inclusive and unbounded feeling of unity and association.

NOTES

Chapter 9:
Practical Guide to Applying the Polyvagal Theory

S tanley Rosenberg focuses on the basic intricacies of our lives as individuals and as a society in general. It is not because life is changing more than it has in the past, but the world seems to be going into a stranger form of existence, whereas we try to fix one problem, and it can lead to several unintended outcomes. This makes more grounded people live in anxiety, especially those trying to overcome an overwhelming trauma.

People who work with others going through trauma might need to proceed more slowly, as it is understood that the trauma in a person's body partly exists because the body has refused to let it go.

Stephen Porges developed the polyvagal theory, which looks at the nervous system and exactly how it responds to stress and danger. It is often described as a 3-part hierarchical system, and as the theory describes, the body assesses stress or danger through certain signals from the environment. Basically, if we begin to perceive stress, sooner or later, sympathetic activation comes into play.

The way the brain is wired has not changed much over time. It is designed to protect us from dangers of various forms either by fight or by flight, by activation, or by deactivation. When we encounter danger, the social engagement system is stimulated first; if we find that it doesn't do the trick, our activation system engages. That means we are ready to jump into action, and our heart rate starts increasing. If the threat gets too large to be managed, the body activates the dorsal vagus system as a last resort. This theory can be applied in various situations, as described in the following section.

Anxiety

Anxiety is the body's natural response to stress, and many people experience anxiety from time to time, but that doesn't necessarily mean they have an anxiety disorder. This is because anxiety is basically the feeling of apprehension or even fear of future events. People can become anxious in different places and for different reasons. It could occur because of a job interview or a speech or even the first day of school, either as a student or as a teacher. These make the brain and the mind more fearful and nervous.

It is well known that anxiety and panic attacks have an impact on blood pressure and that the vagus nerve connects to various organs in the body. When an organ is not stimulated by the vagus nerve, it can lead to issues ranging from anxiety to stomach-related problems.

Less stimulated or unstimulated vagus nerve branches could be a leading cause of anxiety and panic attacks.

Let's use this example: if your anxiety's root cause is a stomach issue, then when your vagus nerve is stimulated, your vagal tone increases, helping your stomach and solving your anxiety issue. Now you might be wondering exactly how to increase your vagal tone. There are many activities known to increase vagal tone and activation, and they range from breathing exercises to singing, etc. Although these are fantastic methods for stimulation of the vagus nerve, the best method is through the use of cold therapy/ice.

This is a very practical way of relieving yourself of anxiety using the polyvagal theory. When you expose your vagus nerve to cold conditions, it tends to shut down the body's fight-or-flight response to feelings such as anxiety and panic attacks. For example, placing an ice pack at the back of the neck is sure to boost your parasympathetic nervous system. This calms a person down almost immediately as it reduces the heart rate.

Ice packs aren't the only thing that can be used, as even a cold shower or using ice-cold water on your face accompanied by deep breaths can calm your anxiety.

So next time you feel your anxiety rising or feel a panic attack coming on, go to the freezer and get an ice pack and place it gently at the back of your neck, and don't forget to take deep breaths. In doing so, you'll be able to sense your body calming down.

Depression

The polyvagal theory can be applied to depression in different ways. To understand it better, we have to look at the visceral level of vagal nerve activation through this theory. Mental disorders such as depression are mostly caused by the malfunctioning of the autonomic/vegetative nervous system. Both the parasympathetic and sympathetic systems are dominant, while the vagal tone is low. In depression, there is a constant level of stress which makes a person consistently feel uneasy and prevents them from behaving appropriately.

This is why people suffering from depression lack the passion and drive for many things and are unable to relax. Their sleep is unrefreshing, and they tend to wake up tired. In depression, the "smart vagus" (ventral vagus) system cannot cope with the sympathetic branch of the nervous system.

Naturally, after a stressful experience, the "smart vagus" should be able to enforce a "vagal brake" (vagal stimulation) or sympathetic deactivation, decreasing the heart rate and stabilizing the breathing pattern. However, this action can be blocked by traumatic experiences, and this leads to imbalance. So instead of smart vagus activation, the parasympathetic replaces the sympathetic, and this can lead to apathy in a person.

Breathing exercises are a great way to heal depression for various reasons. The key functions of the autonomic nervous system include regulating heart rhythm as well as breathing. These are both controlled by the vagus nerve. Breathing is relaxed and calm when the smart (ventral) vagus is active, while the sympathetic system handles breathing when under stress by causing shorter and shallower breaths.

When you learn to improve your breathing, you can access the vagal brakes (vagal activation causing sympathetic deactivation). People battling depression would need to change several aspects of their breathing, including taking deeper breaths in order to expand their lung capacity and to increase oxygen metabolism. There are additional benefits to taking deeper breaths, such as building one's self-esteem, confidence, and trust in themselves.

Also, note the quality of the exhale because it also affects the sympathetic system. A relaxed breath doesn't just fill your lungs with oxygen, but it comes with acceptance and trust. Breathing therapy is a good way to let go of all obstacles to focus on achieving relaxed breathing. By doing so, you are letting go of the trauma that causes the failure of the vagal brake. Breathing exercises can help in restoring balance by accessing and healing the vagal brake.

Although this could seem like a stressful way of handling depression, progress is made with each relaxed, deep breath which helps you on your path to recovery in everyday life.

Trauma

People who have unresolved trauma or PTSD from an event in the past may pass through life in a version of constant fight-or-flight. The main challenge with this is that it disrupts your everyday life and affects your daily activities. There are, however, ways to channel this fight-or-flight response into other activities that can be soothing and relaxing.

Activities such as cleaning the house, working out in the gym, going on a run, or gardening, for example, are great channels, but they might feel different if done with the intention of engaging the social engagement system. However, this can be difficult for some trauma victims as their fight-or-flight sensations cannot be channeled effectively. This causes the body to shut down and make them feel trapped.

If you feel depressed, shut down, and dissociative because of trauma, getting in touch with your fight-or-flight response could prove positive. A good way is through body awareness techniques which are a part of cognitive-behavioral therapy (CBT) and dialectical behavior therapy (DBT). These therapies can help you slowly move away from your shutdown or dissociative responses and become more engaged.

Shutdown responses can be eradicated by understanding your body and becoming more present while being able to attend to momentary muscular tension. Mind and body therapies help in a wide range of areas in health and well-being.

These therapies can help reactivate a person out of shutdown and can encourage the shifting to fight-or-flight responses. Both CBT and DBT help teach individuals to assess their safety better. There is a possible link to feeling safe enough and moving into social engagement activation.

Some of the physical symptoms of trauma include tightness in the chest, exhaustion, and a sinking feeling in the stomach, among others. Massage, tai chi, acupuncture, and counseling, for example, are great mind and body therapies that make us feel more in control and calm.

Autism

The polyvagal theory offers a good explanation for most common autistic features such as social difficulties, sensory sensitivity, and gut dysfunction while at the same time proposing strategies to ease the severity of certain features.

Due to the evolution of mammals, parts of the autonomic nervous system came to be integrated with neural pathways that have control over the face and the head. This makes the ANS a great asset to the control and regulation of senses other than the two common ones. This new circuit is very relevant to the polyvagal view on autism as it can inform more primitive circuits and has also evolved to enable prosocial behaviors.

The vagal pathway also involves a new system that originates in a part of the brain stem, and this helps in controlling muscles of the face and head and also handles facial expressions, speaking, listening, and ingestion. It allows for vocalization and facial expressions, which are powerful approaches to engage in different social behaviors.

When this system is shut down, it results in many of the traits present in autism, such as poor vocal intonation, lack of facial expressions, hypersensitivity to sound, gut problems, defensive stares, and selective eating, among others.

Just as humans are social animals and look at trusted people for safety cues, it may be more difficult for autistic people who neither recognize nor respond to these cues. This is why their bodies detect danger in social engagements.

Transcutaneous vagus nerve stimulation is one way of working with autism. This is a technique whereby an electrical current is applied to the vagus nerve. This nerve runs between the brain and different areas of the body like the heart, the skin, and the gastrointestinal tract. As previously mentioned, the vagus nerve is very important to both the physical and emotional responses in the body and enters either fight-or-flight mode or rest-and-digest.

The vagus nerve can be stimulated electrically through an implanted device or an external device applied to the skin. If you think this sounds dangerous, you should know that vagus nerve stimulation is an FDA-approved treatment for seizures, and research has shown that this same treatment can be used for depression.

Different research studies have shown that when treated with thoracic vagus nerve stimulation (TVN), children with autism have shown improvement in their behaviors, cognitive functions, and, of course, seizure frequency.

How to Optimize Your Autonomic Functioning Using the Polyvagal Theory

During the last trimester in utero and the following year after birth, the autonomic nervous system undergoes rapid changes. These changes are necessary so infants can breathe, maintain body temperature, obtain food, and much more. Such development is the basic progression in the biology of infants to regulate their physiological and behavioral state when interactions with another person take place, which is most likely the mother at first.

It is thought that these developmental changes and their neural pathways, which regulate the autonomic state, can provide a neural platform in supporting the abilities of infants to be expanded when they engage with objects as well as people in a frequently changing environment. This causes the emerging behavioral patterns and social interaction needs and desires of a growing infant to be viewed within the context of maturational alterations in their autonomic nervous system.

Since the autonomic nervous system plays a crucial role in a child's survival when they transition from the prenatal to the postnatal environment, it is quite astonishing that the central mechanisms of the autonomic nervous system have been digressive to pediatric medicine.

The nervous system of mammals did not just develop for the sole purpose of surviving in life-threatening and dangerous situations but also to promote social interactions and bonding. To achieve this adaptive flexibility, a new neural strategy seeking safer environments has been developed while the more primitive neural circuits regulating defensive approaches have been retained. To accommodate both fight-or-flight as well as social engagement behaviors, the modern vagal system in mammals has evolved to enable rapid, adaptive shifts in more autonomic situations.

Three Organizing Principles

There are 3 organizing principles when it comes to the polyvagal theory, namely hierarchy, neuroception, and co-regulation.

Hierarchy

The autonomic nervous system responds to sensations in the body and signals from the environment with one of 3 different responses. These pathways are activated in a particular order, the order of evolution when it comes to responding to challenges predictably. They include the dorsal vagal branch, which has to do with immobilization, the sympathetic nervous system for mobilization, and lastly, the ventral vagus branch, which is in charge of social engagement and connection.

Neuroception

This is a word coined by Dr. Porges himself, which he used in describing the various ways the autonomic nervous system responds to people or situations that appear safe, dangerous, or life-threatening situations.

Co-regulation

Co-regulation describes how an individual's responses are influenced by the responses of another person. The polyvagal theory identifies co-regulation as an important biological response as it is viewed as necessary to sustain life. Through this reciprocal regulation of various autonomic states, we decide whether we feel safe enough to want a connection and create and sustain certain relationships. The autonomic nervous system is thought of as a foundation upon which all life experiences are built. It is viewed as the platform upon which we base all our experiences. The various movements we make in the world, such as connecting and isolating, coming and going, etc., are all directed by the ANS.

With supportive, co-regulating relationships, we tend to become much more resilient. These relationships help us master the art of survival, and that is why the ANS is continually learning habits of creating connection and protection in relationships.

It is hopeful to say that early intervention can help shape the nervous system, as can ongoing experiences. As we know, the brain continuously adapts our responses to different environments and experiences. The ANS is very engaged, and we, too, can influence it as we please. Our nervous system is built to reach out for co-regulation as we experience moments of either safety or danger. The signals conveyed, either of safety or of danger, which are sent from one autonomic nervous system to another, can regulate or increase certain reactions.

Optimizing Autonomic Function

Optimizing your autonomic functioning can be done through taking deep breaths, box breathing, cold/ice, and gut health.

Deep Breathing

Although this might seem cliché, there is a connection between respiration and heart rate, which affects the vagus nerve. This is a good reason why yoga can help reduce overall stress. Breathing exercises can increase vagal tone and help in managing blood pressure.

Box Breathing

When having a panic attack, you can try box breathing as follows:

Inhale and count to 4

Hold and count to 4

Exhale and count to 4

Wait and count to 4

You can repeat these steps until you are in control again.

The reason this helps is that the slow expansion of your lungs can send signals to slow down your heart, and this can help calm your entire body, including your nervous system. The vagus nerve connects the signaling and releasing of acetylcholine which is a calming chemical that helps the body relax.

Remember the Cold?

Never forget that cold tunes the vagus response, and this can slow down sympathetic nervous system activation. Cold exposure can help in relieving depression and anxiety. When you stimulate the vagal pathway, you also stimulate digestion. Cold exposure can reactivate the gastric nerves.

Take Care of Your Gut

Did you know that microorganisms in the digestive system communicate with the brain? The microbiome can be said to be the ecosystem of good bacteria present in your body and on your skin. Most times, when people talk about this, they are referring to the microbes in the colon and intestines.

There have been studies on animal models as well as some human evidence that when the microbiome is thriving, it can boost mood and reduce anxiety. To determine if the vagus nerve was the reason for this, experiments were conducted on rodents with and without a vagus nerve. The ones with the vagus nerve seemed to experience reductions in anxiety as well as depression indicators, unlike those without.

Developing Your Child

As a parent, you can help build the autonomic system of your child and tune their vagal pathways through loving care and bonding.

Giving your kids cold showers shouldn't be the first step, as you should wait until they know that's what they want. During the infant stage, baby massages and skin-to-skin contact can help develop the baby's vagal tone. Once children are older, other ways to help tone their vagus nerve are cold blast showers and breathing techniques. Other ways to develop this include yoga, massage, and mind-body techniques. The benefit of toning the vagus nerve is that it extends to the major organs in the body.

Surgically Implanted Electrical Vagus Nerve Stimulator

The vagus nerve can be activated surgically in order to more aggressively treat a dysfunction. There are surgical implants to stimulate the vagus nerve, such as electric stimulators for patients who suffer from severe epilepsy or depression.

Find Your Safety Cues and Train Them

Finding your safety cues and training them with a little practice can help you feel safe. Your safety cues can keep your anxiety and fear responses from kicking in. A good way to go about this is finding your safe place or your happy place when you are calm. To do this, imagine you are in the place you feel most at ease and peaceful. Ensure to make use of sensory information as much as possible such as smells, sounds, and sights, and practice this visualization often. Then when you begin to experience fear or anger, you can initiate your safe place visualization with little effort.

NOTES

Conclusion

The polyvagal theory has had a global impact on both clients and counselors; many counselors have used this theory to improve many health statuses. Many of the things stated help us in facing the reality of life, including putting a smile on our faces, dancing out stress, singing, playing an instrument, having a correct state of thought, being among positive people, knowing how to control your body to not enter into trauma and reaching out to a counselor. All these are very true to help everyone in any kind of distress. Based on this theory, Porges has been able to break down music therapy into behavioral processes to encourage social engagement into action and to find out how clients react behaviorally and physiologically.

When calm, there is a physiological regulation in our behavior. We have also learned that a mechanical change in our breathing has an increase in the influence of calming and a good health benefit to the vagus nerve. This has helped in reducing the number of health attacks we had back then. Also, try from now on to be positive once finished with this book. Don't ever say, "it will never work" or "I can't." When we change all these thoughts, sooner or later, you will appreciate the theory. Try to always look out for neighbors who have a similar problem to the ones stated and help them out with this exercise; it could also be a practical way to see how the polyvagal theory works. It is also important to keep records as a client on how it has changed your health.

The normal functioning of the body is regulated by what Stephen Porge calls the "Social Engagement System" (social communication). This vagus system enables us to interact and communicate with other people from birth. But when we are stressed, it diminishes our ability to do that.

He/she should take advantage of breathing exercises. Since the vagus is active when the breaths are calm and the sympathetic system is active when the breaths are distorted, short and shallow breaths tend to create a form of imbalance in the nervous system. Depressed people should learn to change their breathing habits by taking longer inhales to stretch the capacity of the lungs to take in more oxygen and longer exhales for relaxation.

For autistic people, while growing up, their body system was immobilized. The consequence is that they became agitated, have difficulties digesting food, and their interactions with the outside community are distorted.

So there is a beautiful ray of hope for autistic patients. Through several therapies and counseling sessions, people suffering from autism can learn to reconnect with their brain and body, gain mastery over it, and above all, feel safe and secure in this beautiful world of ours.

To give you the needed time to digest all the information you've absorbed from this book, I will end my tirade here. I hope this book has taught you all you need to know about the polyvagal theory.

NOTES